# PCOS:

*An Informative Guide on Living with Polycystic Ovary Syndrome*

I0468560

by
Mary
Criswell-Carpenter

DISCLAIMER

*The information provided herein is stated to be truthful and consistent, in that any liability, in terms of inattention or otherwise, by any usage or abuse of any policies, processes, or directions contained within is the solitary and utter responsibility of the recipient reader. Under no circumstances will any legal responsibility or blame be held against the publisher for any reparation, damages, or monetary loss due to the information herein, either directly or indirectly. Respective authors hold all rights not held by publisher.*

Other books by
Mary Criswell-Carpenter available on
Amazon.com

## Fiction

<u>Maggie and the Stubborn Swede</u>
<u>Mary and the Marauding Indians</u>
<u>Katy and the Wolves at the Door</u>

## Non-Fiction

<u>Turmeric: The Natural Pain Reliever for
Arthritis and So Much More..</u>

This book is dedicated to the brave women in
my family living with
PCOS,
and especially,

*Shelby*

# Table of Contents

# Introduction

Thank you for downloading **PCOS: *An Informative Guide on Living with Polycystic Ovary Syndrome.***

In this book we teach you the basics:
- What Is PCOS?
- What Causes PCOS?
- What are the Symptoms of PCOS?
- Does Having Ovarian Cysts Mean that I have PCOS?
- Can PCOS Increase the Risk of Other Diseases?
- Diabetes and PCOS
- High Blood Pressure and PCOS
- Obesity and PCOS
- Heart Disease, Stroke and PCOS
- Cancer and PCOS
- How is PCOS Diagnosed?
- What is the Purpose of all these Tests?
- How is PCOS Treated?
- Pharmaceutical Remedies
- Can I Treat PCOS at Home?
- Does PCOS Affect Fertility?
- Current Medical Research on PCOS
- Vitamin D Deficiency Common in PCOS

- Increase in the Development of Anxiety and Depression in PCOS
- Higher Levels of Cholesterol, Triglycerides Associated with PCOS after 50
- Nonalcoholic Fatty Liver Disease Associated with PCOS

We discuss each issue and the ramifications and complications associated with Polycystic Ovary Syndrome.

If you or a family member suspect you have this disease, download this book now for an Informative Guide to Living with Polycystic Ovary Disease.

# Chapter One: A Personal Experience with PCOS

My name is Shelby. I am 22 years old and I was diagnosed PCOS in March 2013, about 3 years ago. I was 15 when I first started developing ovarian cysts. I would get them every few months and they were very painful.

For two years, my general practitioner told me developing cysts was normal for teenagers. When I was 17, I ended up going to a different doctor for my many health problems. This doctor believed my cysts were caused by my birth control pills, which had been prescribed to help regulate my menstrual cycle.

I had always experienced heavy, painful, and irregular menstrual cycles. Birth control pills had been the only solution to make them regular. This doctor advised me to stop taking the birth control pills and instead prescribed a non-hormonal based birth control.

This doctor also told me she did not believe I would ever be able to become pregnant because of the damage to my ovaries. Eight weeks later I found out I was pregnant.

After my pregnancy, my body begin to experience more health problems. I stopped having menstrual cycles altogether. I would become violently ill in the morning, as if I had a severe case of morning sickness, even though I wasn't pregnant. I developed severe acne and headaches.

My obstetrician set me up an appointment with a gynecologist in her office. The gynecologist said I could not possibly be experiencing these symptoms since I wasn't pregnant. She did do a test for viruses which came back negative. She chalked up all my symptoms to stress and told me to relax.

When I did not get better, I returned to her with the same diagnosis and this time she prescribed anti-depressants. I decided to get a second opinion.

The next doctor had no idea what would cause my symptoms and began running tests. All of the tests came back negative. I asked her to test me for ovarian cysts because of my history, but she refused. I got frustrated and stopped seeing doctors altogether.

Five months later I got a positive home pregnancy test. For three months, doctors did blood and urine tests which all came up negative. Finally, an ultrasound was ordered which showed multiple ovarian cysts. The doctor did not offer treatment for the cysts but declared the cysts had caused a false positive. She said the cysts should dissolve on their own.

I finally went to a walk in clinic which had a doctor visiting from Germany. She recognized my symptoms immediately. She confirmed with blood tests and diagnosed me with PCOS. She was not able to treat my disease, but made a referral to a fertility specialist since we were trying to conceive. He treated me with metformin, provera, and clomid. I got pregnant on the third round of medications.

I did not suffer from PCOS symptoms during my pregnancy and felt much better about my condition. After my twins were born, I could not stop bleeding, so the fertility specialist put me back on metformin. The metformin made me sick, but he said there was no alternative, so I was left without treatment.

At 9 weeks postpartum, my midwife prescribed birth control pills to help with my bleeding. Later she recommended mirena but the mirena made my symptoms worse. I had it removed after a year. My symptoms continued and I continued to see more doctors.

What I have discovered over the past three years is women with PCOS see one of four doctors most of the time.
1. Doctors who do not treat PCOS at all.
2. Doctors who do not believe PCOS exists.
3. Doctors who treat PCOS with birth control and metformin.
4. Doctors who treat only for fertility reasons.

Another obstacle I have found is that insurance providers consider PCOS a fertility problem only. Many will not cover treatment at all if the diagnosis is PCOS. They consider fertility to be elective instead of necessary treatment.

As for me, I have hit a wall with my PCOS treatment. I can not get a referral to a doctor who will treat PCOS because insurance says they do not cover fertility issues. It has been two years since my twins were born and I have just recently found a natural treatment which helps me.

PCOS has been a struggle for me and many other women who are pushed aside by medical personnel.

# Chapter Two: What Is PCOS?

Polycystic Ovary Syndrome, or PCOS, is a hormonal disorder affecting women of all ages. Symptoms can begin as early as age eleven, but can be present later in life also. PCOS, sometimes referred to as Stein-Leventhal Syndrome, is considered to be one of the most widespread hormonal endocrine syndromes and is considered genetic in nature. The disease is often referred to as a silent killer because it is so hard to diagnosis and can lead to other medical conditions. Instead of one single test to diagnosis PCOS, patients must undergo multiple tests to confirm different symptoms of the disease. (http://www.pcosfoundation.org/what-is-pco)

Without treatment, PCOS can lead to other serious diseases brought about by the hormone imbalance associated with the disease. Hormones are like tiny messengers which send signals throughout the body, so when imbalances occur, those messages are misdirected. The messages include such requests as to produce more hormones which control such things as energy levels and growth. Since many of the messages are to produce more or different hormones, the imbalance negatively affects energy which can lead to other serious health issues.

## What Causes PCOS?

The actual cause of PCOS is not known, other than it is passed down from generation to generation. The disease causes an excessive production of androgens, a male sex hormone women also produce, which is believed to be the underlying problem. The excessive amounts of androgens can prevent ovulation which causes an abnormal menstrual cycle in many women.

One possible cause of passing this disease from generation to generation is the excessive exposure to androgen while in the womb. When the mother suffers from PCOS, releasing an overproduction of androgen, the baby is exposed to those extra hormones during the incubation process. The extreme exposure to androgen for an extended period of time during formation may prevent the genes producing the hormone from ever working correctly.

http://www.obesityaction.org/educational-res ources/resource-articles-2/obesity-related-dise ases/polycystic-ovarian-syndrome-pcos-and-o besity

# Chapter Three: What are the Symptoms of PCOS?

PCOS is very difficult to diagnosis because of the wide range of symptoms which are seemingly unrelated. Probably the most common symptom is the many ovarian cysts associated with PCOS; however, many women do not even realize when a ovarian cyst is present.

With the wide range of symptoms, the disease is difficult to discern. Making diagnosis even harder is the fact that symptoms are never exactly the same for two different women, even when they are relatives. Some women experience excessive hair growth, called hirsutism, while others experience hair loss sometimes resembling male pattern baldness.

Acne can sometimes result from PCOS because of the hormone imbalance, which may be extreme. Acne is a very common condition, especially among adolescents, so acne alone will not likely lead to diagnosis. If the PCOS is undiagnosed, the woman may believe it is just acne and treat it with chemicals with little success.

Hypo- or hyperthyroidism may be a symptom resulting in obesity, sometimes extreme, or conversely, low body weight. Obesity is a growing problem in this country which is highly stigmatized. Many people assume an obese person just simply has no self control, overeating or binge eating instead of controlling their caloric intake. This stigmatism leads to criticism from all levels, including the very doctor meant to treat the disease.

One common symptom for most patients with Polycystic Ovarian Syndrome is low fertility, or sometimes even infertility. This is often the symptom which leads to the PCOS diagnosis. Gynecologists are often trained to recognise the symptoms of PCOS in patients with fertility issues. Unfortunately, many Gynecologists are unwilling to treat patients with PCOS if they are not attempting pregnancy or after pregnancy is achieved.

An Endocrinologist can diagnose and treat PCOS in women without the desire of pregnancy. Since it is not limited to infertility, a woman with a PCOS diagnosis should continue to seek regular treatment at all times.

Here is a list of some other common symptoms:
- oily skin
- skin tags
- obstructive sleep apnea
- dandruff
- Dark patches of skin, usually around the neck, thighs, breasts, and/or arms
- Unexplained pelvic pain
- Depression
- Anxiety

## Does Having Ovarian Cysts Mean that I have PCOS?

No, most women experience ovarian cysts at least once during fertile years. Many cysts are completely harmless and painless, as they go away on their own. When a woman suffers from PCOS, the cysts occur more frequently and often appear in what is referred to as a "string of pearls" formation. (http://www.pcosfoundation.org/what-is-pco)

Not all doctors are trained to recognize this formation of cysts as possibly identifying PCOS. Without the PCOS diagnosis, the doctor might prescribe a hormone based birth control pill. The synthetic hormone meant to correct the underlying hormone imbalance may lead to more cysts. These synthetic hormones may also further exacerbate the hormone imbalance, leading to even more symptoms.

Unfortunately, many women will eventually undergo an unnecessary hysterectomy because of the lack of diagnosis. This is because the hormone imbalance often causes excessive or heavy menstruation. The popular treatment for the heavy menstruation is again birth control pills which intensifies the problem.

# Chapter Four: Can PCOS Increase the Risk of Other Diseases?

Yes, since PCOS is caused by abnormal hormone levels, it does increase the risk of other diseases when left untreated. Diseases such as diabetes, high blood pressure, obesity, stroke, and heart disease can occur as a result of untreated PCOS. In some extreme cases, the untreated PCOS can lead to certain forms of cancer.

https://www.pcos.com/pcos-and-heart-disease-what-are-the-implications/

## Diabetes and PCOS

Women who suffer from PCOS often suffer from insulin resistance. Diabetes is thought to be a disease in which the body does not produce enough insulin to break down the sugar which enters the body. This is actually Type I diabetes, sometimes referred to as

Juvenile Diabetes. There is another kind of diabetes, Type II diabetes, or Adult Onset Diabetes. In the case of Type II diabetes, people are suffering from insulin resistance; the body produces insulin but cannot properly use the insulin it produces. When the body does not use the insulin, the pancreas secretes more insulin, because it has determine it did not produce enough insulin. The excessive insulin resulting from the overproduction causes the ovaries to produce more androgen, which as we learned earlier is the root cause of PCOS.

This condition is often treated with diabetes medications which have little to no effect. They have little to no effect because most diabetes medications provide artificial insulin. Since the insulin resistance does not equal lack of insulin, the added insulin does not help to break down the body's glucose content. Instead, the additional insulin increases belly or abdominal fat, which in turn, creates more insulin resistance and infertility.

There are medications designed to treat insulin resistance, such as metformin or glucophage, by encouraging the body to use the existing insulin. These treatments are often used to treat women with PCOS diagnosis because they do work to lower glucose levels. They are also used to treat infertility which will be discussed in a later chapter.

The insulin resistance allows excessive insulin to travel through the arteries causing damage along the way. This excessive insulin can cause injury to the arterial tissue as well as cause a buildup of plaque in the arteries. A buildup of plaque along the arterial walls is commonly known as atherosclerosis. (https://www.pcos.com/managing-hypertension-high-blood-pressure/)

## High Blood Pressure and PCOS

Women who suffer from PCOS often experience high blood pressure. High blood pressure can affect anyone and usually accompanies obesity or excessive weight gain. The excessive weight gain in women suffering from PCOS is often the result of the insulin resistance, common among sufferers.

The biggest concern with high blood pressure is the long term damage to the heart, which can lead to either a heart attack or stroke. The increased levels of insulin, and therefore increased levels of glucose, can cause a rise in triglyceride levels which can cause plaque. Another concern is that high cholesterol levels resulting from high insulin levels can lead to even more risk of heart disease or stroke. When high blood pressure goes undetected and/or untreated, this risk increases significantly.

According to the National Institute of Diabetes and Digestive and Kidney Diseases high blood pressure causes microscopic damage to the kidneys. The two major causes of kidney failure are:

1. diabetes 43%, and
2. high blood pressure 28%.

Women that have undiagnosed PCOS are at risk of kidney failure from a double causation. (http://www.womenshealth.gov/publications/our-publications/fact-sheet/polycystic-ovary-syndrome.pdf)

## Obesity and PCOS

The insulin resistance common in women with PCOS can lead to weight gain, often to obesity levels. This is because the insulin is used to breakdown glucose in the body. When the insulin does not breakdown the glucose, then both the insulin and glucose buildup in the bloodstream.

The buildup leads to increased levels of androgen hormone in the body. The high androgen levels can cause excessive weight gain, especially in the abdominal region. This increased abdominal fat is often associated with health conditions such as heart disease. A change in diet alone is unlikely to help a woman with PCOS to lose weight. (http://www.webmd.com/women/guide/polyc ystic-ovary-syndrome-pcos-and-weight-gain)

# Heart Disease, Stroke and PCOS

According to Dr. Paul Hardiman, women who suffer from PCOS are almost twice as likely to develop atherosclerosis. The development of atherosclerosis significantly increases the risk of heart disease or stroke.

(https://www.pcos.com/pcos-and-heart-disease-what-are-the-implications/)

# Cancer and PCOS

Untreated PCOS can lead to the development and diagnosis of uterine cancer. Uterine cancer is characterized by the growth of cancer cells within the uterus.

The uterus consists of two linings. The inner lining is called the endometrium. The outer lining is call the myometrium which is a muscular lining.

Adenocarcinoma is the most commonly diagnosed uterine cancer, which begins in the endometrium liner. There is a form of cancer found in the myometrium called sarcomas but it is much less common.

(http://texasstrokeinstitute.com/hl/?/11479/Endometrial-cancer)

# Chapter Five: How is PCOS Diagnosed?

Diagnosis of PCOS is very tricky because there is not one single test available to confirm the disease. A knowledgeable doctor will perform multiple tests and use the combined results to make a diagnosis. The tests will include an ultrasound, a blood test, a physical exam, a pelvic exam, and an examination of the patient's medical history.

## What is the Purpose of all these Tests?

The ultrasound is performed to determine if there are any ovarian cysts and the thickness of the uterus. Ovarian cysts were discussed in chapter 2 covering symptoms. What does the thickness of the uterus have to do with PCOS? Excessive estrogen is a common cause for thickness of the uterus. Since PCOS is a hormone imbalance, then excessive thickness could be a sign of too much estrogen. The doctor may also request a endometrial biopsy to look for cancer or precancerous cells. Again, not all women will experience either or all of these symptoms, so the tests can not be limited to only an ultrasound. (http://obgyn.ucla.edu/body.cfm?id=330)

The blood test is used to test several different levels which are commonly abnormal in PCOS patients.

- HCG - HCG levels are tested to verify the patient is not pregnant. Since pregnancy affects hormone levels, it would be very difficult to positively identify PCOS in a pregnant patient.
- Testosterone - Testosterone is an androgen, so high levels would help to identify a hormonal imbalance. High levels of testosterone in women lead to such symptoms as hair loss, acne, facial hair commonly associated with men, and irregular menstrual cycles.
- Prolactin - Prolactin is a hormone made by the pituitary gland which causes lactation in pregnant women. High prolactin levels in a non-pregnant

women causes irregular menstrual cycles which can lead to infertility.

- Cholesterol and triglycerides - High cholesterol and triglyceride levels can be associated with insulin resistance.
- TSH - TSH, thyroid stimulating hormone, can help to identify either overactive thyroid or underactive thyroid.
- Adrenal hormones - Abnormal adrenal hormone levels can emulate PCOS. The most commonly tested are DHEA-S and 17-hydroxyprogesterone.
- Insulin resistance - insulin resistance is tested by measuring insulin levels and tolerance to glucose. Since insulin resistance is very common in PCOS patients, this test is commonly performed in order to diagnose PCOS. (http://www.webmd.com/women/tc/polycystic-ovary-syndrome-pcos-exams-and-tests)

The physical exam is done to identify visible signs of abnormal hormone levels. The doctor will looks for common symptoms such as excessive hair loss, abnormal facial hair, or acne. Since high blood pressure is a common symptom of PCOS, getting an accurate check of blood pressure can help to identify the disease.

The pelvic exam is done to feel for abnormal thickness in the uterine lining.

The examination of medical history will hopefully help the doctor to determine how long the condition has persisted. Just because a woman has high blood pressure does not automatically mean she has PCOS.

# Chapter Six: How is PCOS Treated?

## Pharmaceutical Remedies

Physicians treating PCOS may choose to treat the many symptoms of the disease with a combination of pharmaceutical remedies and lifestyle changes. The lifestyle changes should be implemented first for a period of time to determine if medication is still necessary. (http://www.womenshealth.gov/publications/our-publications/fact-sheet/polycystic-ovary-syndrome.html)

Since women suffering from PCOS are often overweight, a healthy diet and exercise are an important beginning to treating PCOS. The diet limiting processed foods, as well as sugar intake, is necessary because of the insulin resistance commonly associated with PCOS. A blood test can be performed to determine if the patient suffers from insulin resistance. A goal of losing at least 10 percent of your body weight can help to stabilize blood sugar and hormone levels.

In addition to supplements, it might be helpful to strategically plan your daily calories. Eating the majority of sugar related calories in the morning may help keep glucose levels at a healthy number. The body has all day to digest the sugars since sleep hinders digestion. Try to allow at least 3 to 4 after eating before bedtime.

Decreasing the number of foods with higher levels of AGEs, advanced glycation end products, may also help with the symptoms of PCOS. When glucose is bound to proteins then AGEs are formed. Cutting down on foods which contain higher levels of these compounds, such as processed foods or animal based foods, can help to reduce insulin levels.

High blood pressure poses a serious health risk and is common in women suffering from PCOS. It is usually treated with pharmaceuticals as well as dietary changes. There are a number of pharmaceutical remedies available to treat high blood pressure which fall into different categories.

- Diuretics - diuretics help to expel excess water and sodium thus lowering blood pressure.
- ACE inhibitors, called Angiotensin-converting enzyme - ACE inhibitors prevent the formation of the hormone angiotensin. By preventing angiotensin formation, the blood vessels are allowed to widen so the blood flows freely. Examples are Lisinopril or Ramipril.
- Angiotensin II receptor blockers - These prevent the action of the angiotensin instead of blocking their production. Examples are Valsartan and Losartan.
- Beta blockers - beta blockers block the signals from the hormones and certain nerves sent to the heart and blood vessels. Examples are Atenolol and Metoprolol.
- Calcium channel blockers - These cause relaxation in the cells by preventing calcium from entering the heart and blood vessels. Examples are Nifedipine and amlodipine.
- Renin inhibitors - Aliskiren works to slow down the enzyme called renin from being produced in the kidneys. Renin is

responsible for starting a chain reaction which increases blood pressure.

One of these treatments may not be enough to lower blood pressure to a safe level so your doctor may prescribe a combination of medications. Most doctors will recommend adding one treatment at a time, then allowing time for the body to acclimate to the medication before adding addition treatments. Repeated testing of blood pressure levels may be necessary to determine which treatment is most effective in each individual. (http://www.mayoclinic.org/diseases-conditions/high-blood-pressure/in-depth/high-blood-pressure-medication/art-20046280)

The hormone related symptoms are commonly treated with birth control pills. They may help to regulate menstrual cycles as well as hair growth. Birth control pills are not always tolerated in women with PCOS because they are adding more hormones to an already hormone overloaded body. When they do work, they are only effective when taken every day.

High triglycerides can be treated using pharmaceuticals, such as Lipitor, which works to reduce plaque build up. Dietary changes may also be necessary to control triglycerides.

Insulin resistance is usually treated with pharmaceuticals designed to treat diabetes. Metformin, or glucophage, is commonly used because it works to help the body use the insulin it already produces. Metformin also helps to lower testosterone production.

Infertility will be discussed in a later chapter.

Treating heart disease associated with PCOS is very important and must be treated from several directions. Reducing high blood pressure, triglycerides, cholesterol, and insulin resistance are vital steps but not enough. The doctor will also want to work towards a healthy weight and a balanced diet.
http://www.thelaboroflove.com/articles/how-do-polycystic-ovaries-cause-high-blood-pressure

Women suffering from PCOS often expect menopause to lessen their symptoms since they no longer need to ovulate. This is not the case since irregular menstrual cycles are the result of the disease not the cause. A woman diagnosed with PCOS should continue to receive treatment even after menopause.

# Chapter Seven: Can I Treat PCOS at Home?

Since it is so hard to find a doctor willing to treat PCOS, many women will attempt to treat the symptoms at home. Alternative remedies may offer some relief and can be very effective when taken responsibly. Alternative remedies are not meant to replace a medical treatment.

Alternative remedies include many herbs and minerals available at health food stores and online. Here is a list of some of the common treatments and what they treat. Do not attempt to take them all together but rather one at a time to see how your body reacts to each supplement. Take each for several days before changing supplements or dosage.

- Calcium - Helps to lower testosterone levels.
- Inositol - Inositol is part of the vitamin B family, commonly referred to as B8. Vitamin B8 is important to help prevent the buildup of fatty tissue in the heart and liver, it helps to promote hair growth, it helps to turn nutrients into

usable energy, and it also helps with nerve transmissions. Vitamin B8 is a vital nutrient for the brain and it assists in energy conversion. Energy conversion is vital to women suffering from PCOS because this helps to prevent or at least alleviate insulin resistance by converting glucose to energy. (http://www.onlineholistichealth.com/supplements-2/vitamins/vitamin-b8-inositol.html)

- Vitamin D - Helps to maintain hormone balance and decreases depression.
- N-acetylcysteine - N-acetylcysteine, or NAC, is commonly used for the treatment of infertility in women and shows promise in treating PCOS. NAC is an amino acid as well as an antioxidant. Amino acids are the building blocks for protein. NAC is used by the body in the production of glutathione, which helps to protect the body from free radicals. NAC also reduces insulin buildup in the body which is important in somebody suffering from insulin resistance. (http://www.pcosnutrition.com/links/blogs/nac-and-pcos.html)

- Cinnamon - cinnamon is highly recommended for people suffering from diabetes because it can improve insulin sensitivity. This is also helpful in women suffering from PCOS because of the associated insulin resistances.
- Chromium - chromium is another supplement which can help to decrease insulin resistance by improving the body's sensitivity to insulin.
- B-vitamins - B-vitamins are recommended to women suffering from infertility. These vitamins assist the liver to convert hormones into substances that can be excreted thus removing some of the excess hormones created by women suffering from PCOS. (http://www.marilynglenville.com/womens-health-issues/polycystic-ovary-syndrome/)
- Milk Thistle - milk thistle assists the liver by promoting the healing of cells and to protect against further damage.
- Magnesium - magnesium may improve insulin sensitivity
- Saw Palmetto - saw palmetto has been used to treat prostate problems for a long time because is helps to correct

hormone imbalances. One of the hormones it helps to regulate in the body is androgen. Since androgen is believed to be the primary cause of PCOS, this herb can be very helpful in relieving symptoms and treating the underlying problem.

- Agnus castus - agnus castus helps to normalize pituitary function. It will stimulate the pituitary gland when necessary and also help to control the release of luteinising hormone (LH).
- Black cohosh - black cohosh also helps with the release of LH by reducing the production of the hormone.
- Red Raspberry Leaf - red raspberry leaf helps to regulate the hormones produced in the body.
- Flaxseed - flaxseed will help to reduce the androgen levels in the body because it contains lignans. Lignans cause an increased production of globulin (SHBG), which is a sex hormone that will bind to testosterone in the blood. Flaxseed also works to decrease cholesterol levels by slowing down glucose metabolism. This high fiber supplement contains omega-3 which

reduces inflammation and lowers blood pressure. Omega-3 also helps to lower testosterone levels. (http://www.onemedical.com/blog/live-well/pcos-treatment/)

- Spearmint tea - spearmint tea is another way to decrease androgen levels. It works to reduce testosterone levels while increasing luteinizing hormone and follicle-stimulating hormone levels. By stabilizing these hormones, spearmint tea will help reduce excess body hair called hirsutism.

- Apple Cider Vinegar - apple cider vinegar helps to prevent the body from creating too much insulin and regulate blood sugar levels. By controlling insulin levels, it also helps to control the production of androgens. It may also help with weight loss.

- Fenugreek - fenugreek helps the body to metabolize glucose. Improving glucose metabolism will improve insulin resistance and help to balance hormone levels. This will help to lower cholesterol and aid in weight loss.

- Chasteberry - chasteberry, otherwise known as vitex, helps to balance hormones.
- Fish oil - fish oil is another way to get omega-3 fatty acids and reduce cholesterol levels.
- Licorice root - licorice root helps to reduce testosterone levels by prohibiting the production of an enzyme. The enzyme is necessary for the production of the androgen, testosterone. It also helps to detoxify the liver and aides in ovulation.
- Holy Basil - holy basil is another way to lower androgen levels as well as relieve stress. It has excellent anti-inflammatory and antioxidant properties.
- Turmeric regulates blood sugar levels and is 1,000 times more effective than metformin. It also reduces cholesterol levels.

(http://www.amazon.com/dp/B019ZM8KXC/ref=rdr_kindle_ext_tmb)

Start with one supplement and allow time to ensure the actual affect on your body. Unlike pharmaceuticals, most people do not feel the full effect of a supplement until after they have taken it for several days.

# Chapter Eight: Does PCOS Affect Fertility?

Women with PCOS often suffer from low fertility or even infertility. Unfortunately, many doctors do not even test for PCOS until the woman is unable to become pregnant. General practitioners are not trained to recognize the symptoms and may not even realize PCOS can lead to multiple symptoms. This means the woman has suffered from PCOS for many years without diagnosis or treatment, which leads to more health problems.

Menstrual cycles are often irregular or non-existent because of the abnormal hormones. Once PCOS is diagnosed, there are several treatment options available with a fairly high success rate.

- Clomid - clomid is usually the first fertilization treatment given to women suffering from PCOS. It works by inducing ovulation in women who are not able to ovulate on their own. With Clomid, women 35 and under have a

15% chance of pregnancy. (http://www.advancedfertility.com/clomid-pcos-treatment.htm)

- Metformin - metformin maybe be used with clomid to help stabilize insulin resistance.
- Femara - Femara is another pharmaceutical used to induce ovulation, usually used after clomid fails to cause pregnancy.
- Gonadotropins - gonadotropins are injectable FSH hormones used for 7 to 15 days to help mature the follicle development. There are risks with this treatment including the possibility of multiple births.
- Ovarian drilling - ovarian drilling may be used to reduce the androgen production. A small hole is drilled in an ovary to destroy a portion of the ovary thus reducing the androgen production. (http://www.womenshealth.gov/publications/our-publications/fact-sheet/polycystic-ovary-syndrome.html)
- In-vitro fertilization - when stimulation medications fail, in-vitro fertilization is often recommended to achieve pregnancy. This is a process in which the

egg is fertilized outside of the body then injected into the uterus. (https://www.nichd.nih.gov/health/topics/PCOS/conditioninfo/Pages/infertility.aspx)

PCOS affects the hormones produced by the body. The production of eggs and the preparation of the uterus to receive a fertilized egg can be affected. Not only does it become harder to become pregnant but it is also harder to remain pregnant. If the uterus lining, called the endometrium, is not prepared for the fertilized egg, then miscarriage may result.

(https://www.womentowomen.com/pcos-insulin-resistance/pcos-infertility-answers-to-your-questions/)

# Chapter Nine: Current Medical Research on PCOS

## Vitamin D Deficiency Common in PCOS

There are links between Vitamin D deficits and PCOS, according to research by T. Mahmoudi, M. Sc. at the Department of Genetics at the Royan Institute, Tehran.

A controlled study involving 324 women, half with PCOS and half without, determined that a genetic anamoly in the vitamin D receptor can affect both insulin resistance and PCOS.

**Genetic variation in the vitamin D receptor and polycystic ovary syndrome risk**

Mahmoudi, Touraj

Fertility and Sterility , Volume 92 , Issue 4 , 1381 - 1383

# Increase in the Development of Anxiety and Depression in PCOS

Depression is common for patients with PCOS, according to a study published in Fertility and Sterility, by Dr. E. A. Greenwood. A study involving 301 women determined that PCOS, obesity, and insulin resistance were all common denominators for the increased risk of developing depression after the diagnosis of PCOS.

**Putative role for insulin resistance in depression risk in polycystic ovary syndrome**

Greenwood, Eleni A. et al.
Fertility and Sterility , Volume 104 , Issue 3 , 707 - 714.e1

# Higher Levels of Cholesterol, Triglycerides Associated with PCOS after 50

Hormonal issues do not decline with menopause for the PCOS patient. Studies show that triglyceride levels increase, bad cholesterol increases, testosterone levels and free androgen levels increased for women over 50, far past their child bearing years. This was attributed to an increased risk for cardiovascular disease, stroke and heart attack for women with PCOS. The necessity for proper treatment does not decrease with absence of fertility issues.

### Age-related hormonal and metabolic alterations in women with polycystic ovary syndrome (PCOS)

Panola and Vanky, et al.
Endocrine Abstracts (2013) 32 OC5.3

# Nonalcoholic Fatty Liver Disease Associated with PCOS

Research suggests that women with PCOS have a much higher risk of Nonalcoholic Fatty Liver Disease. Research determined that the women studies had a much higher volume of liver fat, even when taken into account the variables of obesity and insulin resistance. Nonalcoholic

Fatty Liver Disease often has no symptoms until it progresses to liver failure.

**Polycystic Ovary Syndrome with Hyperandrogenism Is Characterized by an Increased Risk of Hepatic Steatosis Compared to Nonhyperandrogenic PCOS Phenotypes and Healthy Controls, Independent of Obesity and Insulin Resistance**

Helen Jones et al.

The Journal of Clinical Endocrinology & Metabolism 2012 97:10, 3709-3716

# Chapter Ten: Conclusion

Thank you again for downloading this book **PCOS:** *An Informative Guide on Living with Polycystic Ovary Syndrome.*

I hope this book was able to help you to learn about the characteristics and challenges of Polycystic Ovary Syndrome.

The next step is to talk with your doctor if you suspect you may have Polycystic Ovary Syndrome. Talk with your relatives also to determine if someone in your family has PCOS, it is a familial disease.

Finally, if you enjoyed this book, please take the time to share your thoughts and post a review on Amazon. It'd be greatly appreciated!

Thank you and good luck!